GET RID OF BARRETT'S ESOPHAGUS: A COMPLETE DIET COOKBOOK

Your Nutritional Roadmap to Symptom Alleviation, Reduced Acid Reflux, and Total Healing from GERD

Audrey McAllister, MD

any such usage must be accompanied by appropriate attribution and citation to the original source.

Requests for permission to use or reproduce any part of this publication should be addressed to the publisher in writing. The publisher reserves the right to grant or deny permission at their discretion, taking into consideration factors such as the intended use, nature of the excerpt, and potential impact on the original work.

Unauthorized reproduction or distribution of copyrighted material is a violation of intellectual property rights and may result in legal consequences. Individuals or entities found to be in breach of copyright law may be subject to legal action, including but not limited to injunctions, damages, and legal fees.

It is the responsibility of all users of this publication to familiarize themselves with and abide by copyright laws and regulations. By accessing or using any part of this work, individuals agree to comply with the terms and conditions set forth by the publisher regarding copyright protection and usage rights.

Table of Contents

FOREWORD

Barrett's esophagus is a condition in which the flat pink lining of the swallowing tube that connects the mouth to the stomach (esophagus) becomes damaged by acid reflux, which causes the lining to thicken and become red.

Between the esophagus and the stomach is a critically important valve, the lower esophageal sphincter (LES). Over time, the LES may begin to fail, leading to acid and chemical damage of the esophagus, a condition called gastroesophageal reflux disease (GERD). GERD is often accompanied by symptoms such as heartburn or regurgitation. In some people, this GERD may trigger a change in the cells lining the lower esophagus, causing Barrett's esophagus.

Barrett's esophagus is associated with an increased risk of developing esophageal cancer. Although the risk of developing esophageal cancer is small, it's important to have regular checkups with careful imaging and extensive biopsies of the esophagus to check for precancerous cells (dysplasia). If precancerous cells are discovered, they can be treated to prevent esophageal cancer.

Who gets Barrett's disease?

In North America, there are about 30 million people who have GERD, the most common long-term gastrointestinal disease. Barrett's esophagus will happen in about 5% of patients with ongoing GERD or esophagus inflammation.

This condition is more common in men than in women and more common in Caucasian

Americans than in African Americans. The average age at diagnosis is 55 years.

Most people with acid reflux don't develop Barrett's esophagus. But in patients with frequent acid reflux, the normal cells in the esophagus may eventually be replaced by cells that are similar to cells in the intestine to become Barrett's esophagus.

SECTION 1: Relationship to Gastroesophageal Reflux Disease (GERD)

Most people who develop Barrett's esophagus have had gastroesophageal reflux disease (GERD) for at least 10 years. But not everyone fits this profile, and other irritants may also lead to Barrett's esophagus.

Causes and Risk factors

What causes Barrett's esophagus?

Scientists don't completely understand why Barrett's esophagus occurs, but it seems to relate to chronic irritation or injury inside your esophagus. It may be a result of constant cellular repair.

The ways that Barrett's esophagus changes your esophagus lining suggest that it's trying to protect itself. Your esophagus lining normally has some protection from acids and other irritants, but not as much as your intestinal lining. Since acids and digestive enzymes do most of their work inside your small intestine, it needs extra protection. Intestinal metaplasia in your esophagus suggests that it does, too.

Factors that increase your risk of Barrett's esophagus include:

Family history: Your odds of having Barrett's esophagus increase if you have a family history of Barrett's esophagus or esophageal cancer.

Being male: Men are far more likely to develop Barrett's esophagus.

Being white: White people have a greater risk of the disease than do people of other races.

Age: Barrett's esophagus can occur at any age but is more common in adults over 50.

Chronic heartburn and acid reflux: Having GERD that doesn't get better when taking medications known as proton pump inhibitors or having GERD that requires regular medication can increase the risk of Barrett's esophagus.

Current or past smoking.

Being overweight. Body fat around your abdomen further increases your risk.

Diagnosis and Tests

How is Barrett's esophagus diagnosed?

A gastroenterologist, a specialist in gastrointestinal diseases, usually diagnoses Barrett's esophagus. They'll look inside your esophagus for evidence of the tissue changes and take small tissue samples to confirm them (biopsies). They'll do this in a procedure called an endoscopy. This means putting a tiny camera on a long tube down your throat to examine your esophagus, while you're under sedation.

What are the signs of Barrett's esophagus on examination?

In general, normal esophageal lining is pale pink and smooth, while intestinal metaplasia is salmon-colored and coarse. But inflammation in your esophagus could obscure these features. Your provider might need to take multiple biopsy samples from different places to study under a microscope. This is how they'll confirm the structural changes in the cells of your esophagus lining (epithelium).

Normal esophageal epithelium consists of stratified squamous cells. These are flat, square cells arranged in layers ("squamous" means flat, and "stratified" means in layers). The lower part of your GI tract (your intestine) is lined with columnar epithelium. Columnar cells are rectangular and lay side-by-side in a single layer. If these appear in your esophagus, your provider will diagnose Barrett's esophagus.

Classifying Barrett's esophagus

Your provider might describe your condition as:

Short-segment Barrett's esophagus. This means the affected area is less than 3 cm long.

Long-segment Barrett's esophagus. This means the affected tissue is longer than 3 cm.

They might define the stage as:

Non-dysplastic metaplasia. This means there's no dysplasia yet and a low cancer risk.

Metaplasia with low-grade dysplasia. This means there's some dysplasia and cancer risk.

Metaplasia with high-grade dysplasia. This means there's significant dysplasia and cancer risk.

Carcinoma. This means dysplasia has progressed to cancer.

Other findings

People with Barrett's esophagus may also have:

Esophageal stricture. This means your esophagus has become narrower, often due to scarring.

Peptic ulcers. These are open sores caused by stomach acid or enzymes.

Symptoms

What are the symptoms of Barrett's esophagus?

On its own, Barrett's esophagus doesn't produce any symptoms. But if something is irritating your esophagus lining for a long time, you're likely to

have symptoms from that. Chronic esophagitis —
inflammation in your esophagus — may feel like
heartburn or chest pain on the lower end, or like a
sore throat if it's higher. It may make your
esophagus feel swollen or cause difficulties
swallowing.

It takes years of chronic esophagitis to damage
your esophagus tissues enough to trigger
metaplasia. If you have any chronic symptoms,
even if they're mild or they come and go, check in
with a healthcare provider. Chronic acid reflux is
the most common cause of esophagitis leading to
Barrett's esophagus. If you ever feel or taste
stomach juices backwashing into your esophagus
after you eat, take notice.

Treatment strategies

Treatment for Barrett's esophagus depends on the extent of abnormal cell growth in your esophagus and your overall health.

No dysplasia

Your doctor will likely recommend:

Periodic endoscopy to monitor the cells in your esophagus. If your biopsies show no dysplasia, you'll probably have a follow-up endoscopy in one year and then every three to five years if no changes occur.

Treatment for GERD. Medication and lifestyle changes can ease your signs and symptoms. Surgery or endoscopy procedures to correct a hiatal hernia or to tighten the lower esophageal sphincter that controls the flow of stomach acid may be an option.

Low-grade dysplasia

Low-grade dysplasia is considered the early stage of precancerous changes. If low-grade dysplasia is found, it should be verified by an experienced pathologist. For low-grade dysplasia, your doctor may recommend another endoscopy in six months, with additional follow-up every six to 12 months.

But, given the risk of esophageal cancer, treatment may be recommended if the diagnosis is confirmed. Preferred treatments include:

Endoscopic resection, which uses an endoscope to remove damaged cells to aid in the detection of dysplasia and cancer.

Radiofrequency ablation, which uses heat to remove abnormal esophagus tissue. Radiofrequency ablation may be recommended after endoscopic resection.

Cryotherapy, which uses an endoscope to apply a cold liquid or gas to abnormal cells in the esophagus. The cells are allowed to warm up and then are frozen again. The cycle of freezing and thawing damages the abnormal cells.

If significant inflammation of the esophagus is present at initial endoscopy, another endoscopy is performed after you've received three to four months of treatment to reduce stomach acid.

High-grade dysplasia

GERD surgery

High-grade dysplasia is generally thought to be a precursor to esophageal cancer. For this reason, your doctor may recommend endoscopic resection, radiofrequency ablation or cryotherapy. Another option may be surgery, which involves removing the damaged part of your esophagus and attaching the remaining portion to your stomach.

Recurrence of Barrett's esophagus is possible after treatment. Ask your doctor how often you need to come back for follow-up testing. If you have treatment other than surgery to remove abnormal esophageal tissue, your doctor is likely to recommend lifelong medication to reduce acid and help your esophagus heal.

Medications

Prescription medications to treat acid reflux include:

Omeprazole.

Lansoprazole.

Pantoprazole.

Rabeprazole.

Esomeprazole.

Dexlansoprazole.

Lifestyle and home remedies

Lifestyle changes can ease symptoms of GERD, which may underlie Barrett's esophagus. Consider:

Maintaining a healthy weight.

Eliminating foods and drinks that trigger your heartburn, such as chocolate, coffee, alcohol and mint.

Stopping smoking.

Raising the head of your bed. Place wooden blocks under your bed to elevate your head.

SECTION 2: Understanding the Link Between Diet and Barrett's Esophagus

Research hasn't shown a significant link between diet and the development or prevention of Barrett's esophagus.

However, if you're dealing with gastroesophageal reflux (GER) or gastroesophageal reflux disease (GERD), adjusting your diet can alleviate or even prevent symptoms. Effective dietary changes may involve:

- Cutting down on fatty foods

- Opting for smaller, more frequent meals rather than three large ones

It's also wise to steer clear of certain foods and drinks that can exacerbate GER or GERD, such as:

- Chocolate

- Coffee

- Peppermint

- Greasy or spicy foods

- Tomatoes and tomato-based products

- Alcoholic beverages

SECTION 3: Dietary Recommendations for Barrett's Esophagus Patients

Anti-Reflux Diet Principles

Following an anti-reflux diet can be helpful in managing symptoms associated with gastroesophageal reflux disease (GERD) or Barrett's esophagus. Here are some key principles to consider:

Avoid Trigger Foods: Certain foods and beverages can worsen reflux symptoms. These typically include acidic or spicy foods, caffeine, chocolate, peppermint, and alcohol. Steering clear of these triggers can help reduce discomfort.

Opt for Low-Fat Foods: Meals high in fat can relax the lower esophageal sphincter (LES), allowing stomach acid to reflux into the esophagus. Choosing low-fat options can help minimize this risk.

Eat Smaller, Frequent Meals: Large meals can increase stomach pressure and lead to more reflux episodes. Eating smaller portions more frequently can prevent this buildup of pressure and reduce the likelihood of reflux.

Stay Upright After Eating: Lying down shortly after a meal can promote reflux by allowing stomach acid to travel back up the esophagus more easily. Remaining upright for at least two to three hours after eating can help prevent this.

Limit Carbonated Beverages: Carbonated drinks can cause bloating and increase stomach pressure, potentially worsening reflux symptoms. Opting for non-carbonated beverages or limiting intake can be helpful.

Watch Meal Timing: Eating too close to bedtime can increase the risk of nighttime reflux. Aim to finish meals at least two to three hours before lying down to sleep.

Raise the Head of Your Bed: Elevating the head of your bed by 6 to 8 inches can help reduce nighttime reflux symptoms by preventing stomach acid from flowing back into the esophagus.

Keep a Food Diary: Tracking your diet and symptoms can help identify specific foods or beverages that trigger reflux. Once identified, you can avoid or limit these items to minimize symptoms.

Stay Hydrated with Water: Water is the best choice for staying hydrated and can help dilute stomach acid. Avoiding excessive consumption of other beverages, especially those that are acidic or caffeinated, can be beneficial.

Foods to Include for Esophageal Health

When it comes to crafting a diet friendly to Barrett's esophagus, certain foods can help alleviate symptoms and promote overall digestive health. Consider incorporating the following options into your meals:

Non-acidic Fruits: Opt for fruits like bananas, melons, apples, and pears, which are less acidic and gentler on the esophagus.

Vegetables: Include plenty of vegetables in your diet, such as leafy greens, broccoli, carrots, and squash. These provide essential nutrients and fiber without aggravating reflux.

Lean Proteins: Choose lean sources of protein, such as skinless poultry, fish, tofu, and beans. These options are easier to digest and less likely to trigger reflux symptoms.

Whole Grains: Incorporate whole grains like oatmeal, brown rice, quinoa, and whole wheat bread into your meals. These grains are rich in fiber and can help regulate digestion.

Dairy Alternatives: If dairy exacerbates your symptoms, try dairy-free alternatives like almond milk, soy milk, or lactose-free dairy products.

Healthy Fats: Include sources of healthy fats, such as avocados, nuts, seeds, and olive oil, in moderation. These fats are beneficial for heart health and may help reduce inflammation.

Herbal Teas: Drink soothing herbal teas like chamomile, ginger, or licorice root tea. These can help soothe the digestive tract and alleviate discomfort.

Water: Stay hydrated with plenty of water throughout the day. Water helps maintain proper digestion and can dilute stomach acid to reduce reflux.

Small, Frequent Meals: Opt for smaller, more frequent meals rather than large ones to prevent excessive pressure on the stomach and reduce the risk of reflux.

Probiotic Foods: Incorporate probiotic-rich foods like yogurt, kefir, sauerkraut, and kimchi into your diet. These foods promote a healthy balance of gut bacteria and support digestive health.

Foods to Avoid or Limit to Alleviate Symptoms

If you're dealing with Barrett's esophagus, certain foods may exacerbate symptoms and should be avoided or limited. Research from a 2017 clinical study suggests that consuming excessive refined sugary foods may heighten the risk of Barrett's esophagus. This occurs because a high-sugar diet can lead to spikes in blood sugar levels, resulting in elevated insulin levels, which in turn may increase the risk of certain tissue changes and cancers.

Additionally, a diet rich in sugar and carbohydrates can contribute to weight gain and obesity.

To minimize these risks, it's wise to cut back on added sugars and simple, refined carbohydrates. This includes avoiding or limiting items like table sugar, glucose, dextrose, maltose, corn syrup, high fructose corn syrup, white breads, flour, pasta, rice, baked goods, boxed cereals, breakfast bars, potato chips, crackers, sugary drinks, fruit juices, soda, ice cream, and flavored coffee beverages.

Furthermore, managing acid reflux through dietary adjustments and other treatments can help prevent worsening of Barrett's esophagus. While trigger foods for acid reflux can vary from person to person, common culprits include fried, spicy, and fatty foods, as well as certain beverages.

Consider limiting or avoiding the following foods if you experience acid reflux or Barrett's esophagus symptoms: alcohol, coffee, tea, milk and dairy, chocolate, peppermint, tomatoes, tomato sauce, ketchup, french fries, battered fish, tempura, onion rings, red meat, processed meats, burgers, hot dogs, mustard, hot sauce, jalapeños, and curries.

However, it's important to note that you don't need to eliminate these foods entirely unless they specifically trigger heartburn or acid reflux symptoms for you. Listen to your body and make adjustments accordingly.

SECTION 4: WHOLESOME RECIPES FOR SYMPTOMS ALLEVIATION

WHOLESOME RECIPES FOR BREAKFAST

Breakfast egg wraps

Ingredients

500g pack closed cup mushrooms

4 tsp rapeseed oil, plus 2 drops

320g cherry tomatoes, halved, or 8 tomatoes, cut into wedges

2 generous handfuls parsley, finely chopped

8 tbsp porridge oats (40g)

10 eggs

4 tsp English mustard powder made up with water

Directions

STEP 1

Thickly slice half the pack of mushrooms. Heat 2 tsp rapeseed oil in a non-stick pan. Add the mushrooms, stir briefly then fry with the lid on the pan for 6-8 mins. Stir in half the tomatoes then cook 1-2 mins more with the lid off until softened.

STEP 2

Beat together the eggs really well with the parsley and oats. Heat a drop of oil in a large non-stick frying pan. Pour in a ¼ of the egg mix and fry for 1 min until almost set, flip over as if making a pancake. Tip from the pan, spread with a quarter of the mustard, spoon a ¼ the filling down the centre and roll up. Now make a second wrap using another ¼ of the egg mix and filling.

Creamy yogurt porridge with apple & raisin compote

Ingredients

For the compote

2 apples, peeled and thickly sliced

25g raisin

150ml orange juice

small handful of sunflower seeds

For the porridge

6 tbsp (50g) porridge oat

300g pot 0% fat probiotic plain yogurt

Directions

STEP 1

For the apple topping: Poach apples in a covered pan with raisins and orange juice for 8-10 mins until the apple is tender. Mash a little of the apple to thicken the juice. Can be made ahead and chilled for up to 1 week. Serve warm or cold on the porridge with sunflower seeds.

STEP 2

For the porridge: Tip 400ml water into a small non-stick pan and stir in porridge oats. Cook over a low heat until bubbling and thickened. (To make in a microwave, use a deep container to prevent spillage as the mixture will rise up as it cooks, and

cook for 3 mins on High.) Stir in yogurt – or swirl
in half and top with the rest.

Date & buckwheat granola with pecans & seeds

Ingredients

For the granola

85g buckwheat

4 medjool dates, stoned

1 tsp ground cinnamon

100g traditional oats

2 tsp rapeseed oil

25g sunflower seeds

25g pumpkin seeds

25g flaked almonds

50g pecan nuts, roughly broken into halves

50g sultanas (without added oil)

For the yogurt & fruit (to serve 2)

2 x 150ml pots low-fat bio natural yogurt

2 ripe nectarines or peaches, stoned and sliced

Directions

STEP 1

Soak the buckwheat overnight in cold water. The next day, drain and rinse the buckwheat. Put the dates in a pan with 300ml water and the cinnamon, and blitz with a stick blender until completely smooth. Add the buckwheat, bring to the boil and cook, uncovered, for 5 mins until pulpy. Meanwhile, heat oven to 150C/130C fan/gas 2 and line two large baking trays with baking parchment.

STEP 2

Stir the oats and oil into the date and buckwheat mixture, then spoon small clusters of the mixture onto the baking trays. Bake for 15 mins, then carefully scrape the clusters from the parchment if they have stuck and turn before spreading out again. Return to the oven for another 15 mins, turning frequently, until firm and golden.

STEP 3

When the mix is dry enough, tip into a bowl, mix in the seeds and nuts with the sultanas and toss well. When cool, serve each person a generous handful with yogurt and fruit, and pack the excess into an airtight container. Will keep for a week. On other days you can vary the fruit or serve with milk or a dairy-free alternative instead of the yogurt.

Vegan tomato & mushroom pancakes

Ingredients

140g white self-raising flour

1 tsp soya flour

400ml soya milk

vegetable oil, for frying

For the topping

2 tbsp vegetable oil

250g button mushrooms

250g cherry tomatoes, halved

2 tbsp soya cream or soya milk

large handful pine nuts

snipped chives, to serve

Directions

STEP 1

Sift the flours and a pinch of salt into a blender. Add the soya milk and blend to make a smooth batter.

STEP 2

Heat a little oil in a medium non-stick frying pan until very hot. Pour about 3 tbsp of the batter into the pan and cook over a medium heat until bubbles appear on the surface of the pancake. Flip the pancake over with a palette knife and cook the other side until golden brown. Repeat with the remaining batter, keeping the cooked pancakes warm as you go. You will make about 8.

STEP 3

For the topping, heat the oil in a frying pan. Cook the mushrooms until tender, add the tomatoes and cook for a couple of mins. Pour in the soya cream or milk and pine nuts, then gently cook until combined. Divide the pancakes between 2 plates, then spoon over the tomatoes and mushrooms. Scatter with chives.

Dippy eggs with Marmite soldiers

Ingredients

2 eggs

4 slices wholemeal bread

a knob of butter

Marmite

mixed seeds

Directions

STEP 1

Bring a pan of water to a simmer. Add 2 eggs, simmer for 2 mins if room temp, 3 mins if fridge-cold, then turn off heat. Cover the pan and leave for 2 mins more.

STEP 2

Meanwhile, toast 4 slices wholemeal bread and spread thinly with butter, then Marmite. To serve, cut into soldiers and dip into the egg, then a few mixed seeds.

Vegan strawberry pancakes

Ingredients

115g wholemeal spelt flour

1 tsp baking powder

1 tsp cinnamon

150ml soya milk

240g soya yogurt

1 tsp vanilla extract

drop of rapeseed oil

200g strawberries, hulled and halved or quartered if large

2 tbsp chopped pecans

a few small mint leaves, optional

Directions

STEP 1

Mix the flour with the baking powder and cinnamon in a bowl using a balloon whisk. In a jug, whisk together the soya milk, 2 tbsp of the yogurt and vanilla extract, then whisk this into the dry Ingredients to make a thick batter.

STEP 2

Rub the oil around the pan using kitchen paper, then set the pan over a medium heat. Spoon in 1½ tbsp batter in three or four places to make small pancakes. Cook over a low heat for 1-2 mins until set, and bubbles appear on the surface, then turn the pancakes using a palette knife. Cook for another 1-2 mins until golden and cooked through. Repeat with the remaining batter to make six pancakes in total.

STEP 3

Serve three pancakes per person topped with the remaining yogurt, berries, pecans and mint leaves.

Peanut butter & banana on toast

Ingredients

2 slices granary bread

1 small banana

½ tsp cinnamon

1 tbsp crunchy peanut butter

Directions

STEP 1

Toast bread and slice banana. Layer banana on one slice of toast and dust with cinnamon. Spread the second slice with peanut butter, then sandwich the two together and eat straight away.

Poached eggs with smoked salmon and bubble & squeak

Ingredients

1 tbsp rapeseed oil

140g white cabbage, finely chopped

2 spring onions, finely sliced

300g whole new potato

1 tbsp snipped chives

2 medium eggs, at room temperature

75g smoked salmon

Directions

STEP 1

Cook the potatoes in a pan of boiling water until tender, then drain.

STEP 2

Heat the oil in a non-stick frying pan or wok. Sweat the cabbage and the spring onions in the pan for a couple of mins. Meanwhile, chop and squash the potatoes roughly, then add to the pan along with the chives. Cook for 4-5 mins, flip it over (don't worry if it breaks) and cook for a further 4-5 mins.

STEP 3

Meanwhile, bring a small pan of water to a rolling boil, then reduce the heat so it is just simmering. Crack the eggs into the pan and simmer for about 3 mins until the whites are cooked and the yolk is just beginning to set. Remove with a slotted spoon and drain on kitchen paper.

STEP 4

To serve, divide the bubble & squeak between 2 plates, place the smoked salmon and poached eggs on top and grind over a little black pepper, to taste.

South American-style quinoa with fried eggs

Ingredients

75g quinoa

400g can black beans, drained

½ tsp ground cumin

½ tsp ground coriander

1 lime, zested and juiced, plus extra wedges to serve

1 tsp cider vinegar

160g cherry tomatoes, halved

1 small avocado, stoned, peeled and roughly chopped

2 tbsp finely chopped coriander

3 spring onions or ½ small red onion, finely chopped

rapeseed oil, for frying

2 medium eggs

Directions

STEP 1

Put the quinoa in a small pan with 250ml water and bring to the boil. Reduce the heat to low, cover and gently simmer for 15-20 mins, stirring occasionally until most of the water has been absorbed and the grains have doubled in size (if there's any water left in the pan, drain well).

STEP 2

Tip into a bowl and stir through the beans, spices, lime zest and juice and vinegar. Stir well, then add the tomatoes, avocado, coriander and onion, and spoon onto plates.

STEP 3

Heat a drop of oil in a non-stick frying pan and fry the eggs until the whites are set with a crispy edge and the yolk is runny. Serve the quinoa topped with the eggs.

Green fritters

Ingredients

140g courgettes, grated

3 medium eggs

85g broccoli florets, finely chopped

small pack dill, roughly chopped

3 tbsp gluten-free flour or rice flour

2 tbsp sunflower oil, for frying

Directions

STEP 1

Squeeze the courgettes between your hands to remove any excess moisture, or tip onto a clean tea towel and twist it to squeeze out the moisture.

STEP 2

Beat the eggs in a bowl, add the broccoli, courgettes and most of the dill, and mix together. Add the flour, mix again and season.

STEP 3

Heat the oil in a non-stick frying pan. Put a large serving spoon of the mixture in the pan, then add 2 more spoonfuls so you have 3 fritters. Leave for 3-4 mins on a medium heat until golden brown on one side and solid enough for you to flip over, then flip over and leave to go golden on the other side. Repeat to make 3 more fritters (there is no need to add any more oil to the pan after the first batch). Scatter with the remaining dill to serve.

Tofu scramble

Ingredients

1 tbsp olive oil

1 small onion, finely sliced

1 large garlic clove, crushed

½ tsp turmeric

1 tsp ground cumin

½ tsp sweet smoked paprika

280g extra firm tofu

100g cherry tomatoes, halved

½ small bunch parsley, chopped

rye bread, to serve, (optional)

Directions

STEP 1

Heat the oil in a frying pan over a medium heat and gently fry the onion for 8 -10 mins or until golden brown and sticky. Stir in the garlic, turmeric, cumin and paprika and cook for 1 min.

STEP 2

Roughly mash the tofu in a bowl using a fork, keeping some pieces chunky. Add to the pan and fry for 3 mins. Raise the heat, then tip in the tomatoes, cooking for 5 mins more or until they begin to soften. Fold the parsley through the mixture. Serve on its own or with toasted rye bread (not gluten-free), if you like.

Buckwheat galettes

Ingredients

80g buckwheat flour

5 medium eggs

250ml milk

2 tsp Dijon mustard

4 tbsp single cream

100g mature gruyère, comté or cheddar, grated

butter, for frying

100g ham, torn

fried mushrooms or steamed spinach, to serve
(optional)

Directions

STEP 1

Mix the flour, 1 egg, the milk and a pinch of salt in
a jug or bowl. Set aside for 30 mins, or up to 3 hrs.
Mash together the mustard, cream and cheese in
another bowl. Heat the oven to 200C/180C
fan/gas 6, and line two baking trays with baking
parchment or foil.

STEP 2

Melt the butter in a large frying pan, then once
foaming, add enough batter to just cover the pan,
swirling it to cover the surface in a thin layer (pour
any excess back into the batter bowl). Cook until
the surface is set and the underside is browning,

carefully flip and cook for another minute or 2, then take off the heat.

STEP 3

Spoon a quarter of the cheese mixture onto the middle of the pancake, using the spoon to create space in the centre to hold an egg. Crack one into the space and lay a few pieces of ham around the edges. Fold each side of the pancake in towards the centre to make a square. Cook in the pan for another 30 secs-1 min, then transfer to a baking tray. Repeat with the rest of the pancakes, then bake for 6-7 mins until the egg whites are set. Serve with fried mushrooms or wilted spinach, if you like.

Almond crêpes with avocado & nectarines

Ingredients

2 large eggs

3 tbsp ground almonds

2 tsp rapeseed oil

1 avocado, halved, stoned and flesh lightly crushed

2 ripe nectarines, stoned and sliced

seeds from 1/2 pomegranate

½ lime, cut into 2 wedges, for squeezing over

Directions

STEP 1

Beat one egg and 1 1 /2 tbsp of the almonds in a small bowl with 1 tbsp water. Heat 1 tsp oil in a large non-stick frying pan over a medium heat and pour in the egg mixture, swirling the pan to evenly cover the base. Cook until the mixture sets and turns golden on the underside, about 2 mins. (There is no need to flip it over.) Turn it out onto a plate and make another one with 1 tbsp water, the remaining egg, oil and almonds.

STEP 2

Top each crêpe with the avocado, nectarines and pomegranate, and squeeze over the lime at the table.

Flatbreads with brunch-style eggs

Ingredients

110g self-raising flour, plus extra for dusting

110g atta or plain wholemeal flour

3 tbsp rapeseed oil, plus extra for the bowl and frying

small knob of butter, melted

For the eggs

1 tbsp olive oil

12 cherry tomatoes, halved

4 large eggs

25g grated cheddar

2 tbsp double cream

Directions

STEP 1

Sift the flours and 1 tsp salt into a large bowl. Add 1 tbsp of the oil and 150ml warm water. Bring together into a soft but not too sticky dough (you may need up to 175ml water). If it feels too wet, add some flour. If it's too dry, add water.

STEP 2

Tip onto a floured surface and knead for 4-5 mins, or until smooth. Put the dough in an oiled bowl, cover and leave for 30 mins.

STEP 3

Tip onto a floured surface. Divide into six balls and roll each out into a thin, 18-20cm wide circle using a rolling pin. If you prefer, you can divide again into twelve balls to make smaller flatbreads.

STEP 4

Brush a heavy-based pan with oil and cook one flatbread over a high heat for 1-2 mins on each side, or until golden and starting to puff. Put on a plate and brush with butter. Repeat with the rest of the dough.

STEP 5

Meanwhile, for the eggs, heat the oil in a small non-stick pan and cook the tomatoes briefly until just softened. Season. Crack the eggs into the pan, add the cheese and cream, cover and cook for 2 mins. Remove the lid. Cook until the egg whites are set, then serve from the pan with the flatbreads, making sure the pan has cooled a little first.

WHOLESOME RECIPES FOR LUNCH

Chunky vegetable soup

Ingredients

2 tbsp rapeseed oil

2 leeks (350g), sliced

3 garlic cloves, finely grated

300g baby potatoes, sliced

1l vegetable stock made with 2 tsp bouillon powder (gluten-free, if needed)

250g asparagus, stems cut into chunks, tips separated

160g baby frozen broad beans or soya beans

400g can borlotti beans, drained

4 tomatoes, chopped

30g pack of basil, stems and leaves separated and finely chopped

For the dumplings

300g tub cottage cheese

75g gram (chickpea) flour, sifted

1 egg, beaten

3 tbsp basil stems and leaves (taken from the 30g in the soup Ingredients above)

Directions

STEP 1

First, make the dumplings. Tip the cottage cheese into a bowl and mash to smooth slightly. Mix in the flour, egg and basil, then set aside for about 10 mins for the flour to absorb the moisture.

STEP 2

Meanwhile, heat the oil in a large pan over a medium heat and fry the leeks, garlic and potatoes for 10-15 mins, or until softened. Pour over the bouillon, then add the asparagus stems, all of the beans, the tomatoes and and remaining basil stems. Bring to the boil, then reduce the heat to a simmer, cover and cook over a medium heat for 10 mins until the veg is tender. Stir in the asparagus tips and remaining basil leaves, and cook a few minutes more. Set aside.

STEP 3

Heat a deep frying pan filled with water to a gentle simmer, then use an ice-cream scoop to scoop eight dumplings into the simmering water. Cook for 5 mins, or until the dumplings rise to the surface.

STEP 4

To serve, divide two portions of soup between bowls and top each with two dumplings. Keep the rest for another day. Will keep chilled in an airtight container for four days. Reheat in a pan for 10 mins over a low heat until piping hot.

Avocado & black bean eggs

Ingredients

2 tsp rapeseed oil

1 red chilli, deseeded and thinly sliced

1 large garlic clove, sliced

2 large eggs

400g can black beans

½ x 400g can cherry tomatoes

¼ tsp cumin seeds

1 small avocado, halved and sliced

handful fresh, chopped coriander

1 lime, cut into wedges

Directions

STEP 1

Heat the oil in a large non-stick frying pan. Add the chilli and garlic and cook until softened and starting to colour. Break in the eggs on either side of the pan. Once they start to set, spoon the beans (with their juice) and the tomatoes around the pan and sprinkle over the cumin seeds. You're aiming to warm the beans and tomatoes rather than cook them.

STEP 2

Remove the pan from the heat and scatter over the avocado and coriander. Squeeze over half of the lime wedges. Serve with the remaining wedges on the side for squeezing over.

Giant couscous salad with charred veg & tangy pesto

Ingredients

2-3 raw beetroot (320g), peeled and chopped

3 red onions (320g), cut into wedges

2 green or orange peppers, deseeded and cubed

1 tbsp olive oil

320g cherry tomatoes

200g wholewheat giant couscous

For the pesto

7g fresh coriander, roughly chopped

15g flat-leaf parsley, roughly chopped

1 garlic clove

1 green chilli, deseeded

½ tsp cumin

1 tbsp apple cider vinegar

1 tbsp olive oil

40g pine nuts, lightly toasted

Directions

STEP 1

Heat the oven to 200C/180C fan/gas 6. In a bowl, toss the beetroot, onions and peppers together with the oil, then spread out on a large roasting tray lined with baking paper and roast for 35 mins. Scatter over the cherry tomatoes, then return to the oven for 10 mins more until the tomatoes have softened and the vegetables are tender.

STEP 2

Meanwhile, cook the couscous following pack instructions, then rinse and drain. To make the pesto, put the coriander and half the parsley in a bowl with the garlic, chilli, cumin, vinegar, oil and 25g of the pine nuts. Add 2 tbsp water, then blitz with a hand blender until smooth or use a small food processor.

STEP 3

Toss the roasted veg and chopped parsley through the couscous and pile on the pesto, then scatter with the remaining pine nuts.

Vegan carbonara

Ingredients

360g wholewheat spaghetti

85g unsalted cashew nuts

2 tsp bouillon powder

2 tsp English mustard powder

1 tsp olive oil

200g baby chestnut mushrooms, halved and thinly sliced

3 garlic cloves, 2 finely grated

1 tsp smoked paprika

2 courgettes (about 320g), peeled then grated

4 tsp nutritional yeast flakes, optional

320g spinach, half cooked each evening as a side dish

Directions

STEP 1

Boil the spaghetti for 10 mins or following pack instructions until al dente, reserving a little of the water. Put the cashews, bouillon and mustard in a bowl, then pour over 350ml boiling water.

STEP 2

Heat the oil in a large non-stick pan. Add the mushrooms and grated garlic, and stir-fry over a high heat until the mushrooms are cooked and starting to crisp up. Take off the heat, stir in the paprika, then tip onto a plate and set aside.

STEP 3

Add the grated courgette to the pan and cook, stirring every now and then until softened. Meanwhile, whizz the soaked cashews, whole garlic clove and nutritional yeast flakes, if using, with a hand blender until completely smooth. Tip the mixture into the pan with the courgettes and briefly stir over the heat.

STEP 4

Add the spaghetti and toss in the cashew and courgette mixture until well coated, then toss through the smoky mushrooms.

Prawn & harissa spaghetti

Ingredients

100g long-stem broccoli, cut into thirds

180g dried spaghetti, regular or wholemeal

2 tbsp olive oil

1 large garlic clove, lightly bashed

150g cherry tomatoes, halved

150g raw king prawns

1 heaped tbsp rose harissa paste

1 lemon, finely zested

Directions

STEP 1

Bring a pan of lightly salted water to the boil. Add the broccoli and boil for 1 min 30 secs, or until tender. Drain and set aside. Cook the spaghetti following pack instructions, then drain, reserving a ladleful of cooking water.

STEP 2

Heat the oil in a large frying pan, add the garlic clove and fry over a low heat for 2 mins. Remove with a slotted spoon and discard, leaving the flavoured oil.

STEP 3

Add the tomatoes to the pan and fry over a medium heat for 5 mins, or until beginning to soften and turn juicy. Stir through the prawns and cook for 2 mins, or until turning pink. Add the harissa and lemon zest, stirring to coat.

STEP 4

Toss the cooked spaghetti and pasta water through the prawns and harissa. Stir through the broccoli, season to taste and serve.

Classic lasagne

Ingredients

2 olive oil, plus extra for the dish

750g lean beef mince

90g pack prosciutto

800g passata or half our basic tomato sauce

200ml hot beef stock

nutmeg

300g fresh lasagne sheets

white sauce

125g ball mozzarella, torn into thin strips

Directions

STEP 1

To make the meat sauce, heat 2 tbsp olive oil in a frying pan and cook 750g lean beef mince in two batches for about 10 mins until browned all over.

STEP 2

Finely chop 4 slices of prosciutto from a 90g pack, then stir through the meat mixture.

STEP 3

Pour over 800g passata or half our basic tomato sauce recipe and 200ml hot beef stock. Add a little grated nutmeg, then season.

STEP 4

Bring up to the boil, then simmer for 30 mins until the sauce looks rich.

STEP 5

Heat the oven to 180C/160C fan/gas 4 and lightly oil an ovenproof dish (about 30 x 20cm).

STEP 6

Spoon one third of the meat sauce into the dish, then cover with some fresh lasagne sheets from a 300g pack. Drizzle over roughly 130g ready-made or homemade white sauce.

STEP 7

Repeat until you have three layers of pasta. Cover with the remaining 390g white sauce, making sure you can't see any pasta poking through.

STEP 8

Scatter 125g torn mozzarella over the top.

STEP 9

Arrange the rest of the prosciutto on top. Bake for 45 mins until the top is bubbling and lightly browned.

Vegan chickpea curry jacket potatoes

Ingredients

4 sweet potatoes

1 tbsp coconut oil

1 ½ tsp cumin seeds

1 large onion, diced

2 garlic cloves, crushed

thumb-sized piece ginger, finely grated

1 green chilli, finely chopped

1 tsp garam masala

1 tsp ground coriander

½ tsp turmeric

2 tbsp tikka masala paste

2 x 400g can chopped tomatoes

2 x 400g can chickpeas, drained

lemon wedges and coriander leaves, to serve

Directions

STEP 1

Heat oven to 200C/180C fan/gas 6. Prick the sweet potatoes all over with a fork, then put on a baking tray and roast in the oven for 45 mins or until tender when pierced with a knife.

STEP 2

Meanwhile, melt the coconut oil in a large saucepan over medium heat. Add the cumin seeds and fry for 1 min until fragrant, then add the onion and fry for 7-10 mins until softened.

STEP 3

Put the garlic, ginger and green chilli into the pan, and cook for 2-3 mins. Add the spices and tikka masala paste and cook for a further 2 mins until fragrant, then tip in the tomatoes. Bring to a simmer, then tip in the chickpeas and cook for a further 20 mins until thickened. Season.

STEP 4

Put the roasted sweet potatoes on four plates and cut open lengthways. Spoon over the chickpea curry and squeeze over the lemon wedges. Season, then scatter with coriander before serving.

Chunky Bolognese soup with penne

Ingredients

2 tsp rapeseed oil

3 onions, finely chopped

3 large carrots, finely diced

2 celery sticks, finely diced

3 garlic cloves, finely chopped

250g pack 5% fat steak mince

500g carton passata

1 tbsp vegetable bouillon powder

1 tsp smoked paprika

4 sprigs fresh thyme

100g wholemeal penne

45g finely grated parmesan, plus extra to serve

Directions

STEP 1

Heat the oil in a large non-stick pan and fry the onions for a few mins. Add the carrots, celery and garlic, then fry for 5 mins, stirring until the vegetables start to soften.

STEP 2

Add the meat and stir well so it breaks down as it cooks. Once it's turned brown, add the passata and bouillon along with 1.3 litres of boiling water. Add the paprika, thyme and some black pepper. Cover the pan and simmer for 15 mins.

STEP 3

Tip in the penne and cook for 12-15 mins until tender. Stir through the cheese, then ladle into bowls. Sprinkle over extra cheese, if you like.

Lentil salad with tahini dressing

Ingredients

2 tbsp cold-pressed rapeseed oil

320g sweet potatoes, cut into cubes

2 large carrots, cut into thin sticks (320g)

2 large courgettes, (375g) cut into chunks

2 medium red onions, halved and sliced

1 tsp cumin seeds

2 tbsp finely chopped ginger

2 tbsp pumpkin seeds

2 x 390g cans green lentils, drained

2 tsp vegetable bouillon powder

1 lemon, zested

good handful of mint, roughly chopped

handful of parsley, roughly chopped

2.5-3 tbsp tahini

1 garlic clove, finely grated

2 x 120g pot bio yogurt

a little smoked paprika, to serve

Directions

STEP 1

Heat the oil in a large non-stick wok. Add the sweet
potato and fry for 5 mins, stirring frequently until

it starts to soften. If it starts to brown too quickly, put a lid on the pan. Add the carrot, courgette, onion, cumin and ginger, then cook over a high heat, stirring frequently, until the veg is tender and a little charred. Stir in the seeds towards the end so they cook for a couple of mins. Remove from the heat and add the lentils, bouillon powder, lemon zest, mint and parsley.

STEP 2

Meanwhile, stir the tahini with the garlic, yogurt and 1 tbsp water to make a dressing. Spoon the lentil salad into bowls and top with the dressing and paprika,

Cumin roast veg with tahini dressing

Ingredients

3 large carrots, roughly chopped

3 peeled raw beetroots, roughly chopped

1 sweet potato, sliced

3 red onions, cut into wedges

250g cauliflower florets

1 tsp cumin seeds

2 tbsp rapeseed oil

1 tbsp balsamic vinegar

2-3 tbsp chopped mint

2-3 tbsp chopped coriander

400g can chickpeas

2 hard-boiled eggs, halved

100g young spinach leaves

For the dressing

3 tbsp tahini

1 tbsp crunchy peanut butter

1 lemon, zested and juiced

1 tsp ground coriander

1 garlic clove, finely grated

Directions

STEP 1

Heat oven to 200C/180C fan/gas 6. Tip all of the vegetables into a large roasting tin. Add the cumin seeds, oil and balsamic vinegar, then toss together. Roast for 45-50 mins until the veg is tender and starting to char.

STEP 2

Meanwhile, mix the tahini and peanut butter with the lemon juice, coriander, garlic and about 4-5 tbsp water to make a dressing.

STEP 3

When the veg is ready, leave to cool a little. Add the mint, coriander, lemon zest and chickpeas, then toss well.

Spicy chicken & avocado wraps

Ingredients

1 chicken breast (approx 180g), thinly sliced at an angle

generous squeeze juice 0.5 lime

½ tsp mild chilli powder

1 garlic clove, chopped

1 tsp olive oil

2 seeded wraps

1 avocado, halved and stoned

1 roasted red pepper from a jar, sliced

a few sprigs coriander, chopped

Directions

STEP 1

Mix the chicken with the lime juice, chilli powder and garlic.

STEP 2

Heat the oil in a non-stick frying pan then fry the chicken for a couple of mins – it will cook very quickly so keep an eye on it. Meanwhile, warm the wraps following the pack instructions or, if you have a gas hob, heat them over the flame to slightly char them. Do not let them dry out or they are difficult to roll.

STEP 3

Squash half an avocado onto each wrap, add the peppers to the pan to warm them through then pile onto the wraps with the chicken, and sprinkle over the coriander. Roll up, cut in half and eat with your fingers.

Summer pistou

Ingredients

1 tbsp rapeseed oil

2 leeks, finely sliced

1 large courgette, finely diced

1l boiling vegetable stock (made from scratch or with reduced-salt bouillon)

400g can cannellini or haricot beans, drained

200g green beans, chopped

3 tomatoes, chopped

3 garlic cloves, finely chopped

small pack basil

40g freshly grated parmesan

Directions

STEP 1

Heat the oil in a large pan and fry the leeks and courgette for 5 mins to soften. Pour in the stock, add three-quarters of the haricot beans with the green beans, half the tomatoes, and simmer for 5-8 mins until the vegetables are tender.

STEP 2

Meanwhile, blitz the remaining beans and tomatoes, the garlic and basil in a food processor (or in a bowl with a stick blender) until smooth, then stir in the Parmesan. Stir the sauce into the soup, cook for 1 min, then ladle half into bowls or pour into a flask for a packed lunch. Chill the remainder. Will keep for a couple of days.

Noodle salad with sesame dressing

Ingredients

For the dressing

1 tbsp sesame oil

2 tsp tamari

1 lemon, juiced

1 red chilli, deseeded and finely chopped

For the salad

1 small onion, finely chopped

2 wholemeal noodle nests (about 100g)

160g sugar snap peas

4 small clementines, peeled and chopped

160g shredded carrots

large handful of coriander, chopped

50g roasted unsalted cashews

Directions

STEP 1

Mix all the dressing Ingredients together in a large bowl, then stir in the onion. Meanwhile, cook the noodles in a pan of boiling water for 5 mins, adding the sugar snap peas halfway through the cooking time – the noodles and peas should be just tender.

Drain, cool under cold running water and drain again. Snip or cut the noodles into smaller lengths to make them more manageable to eat.

STEP 2

Tip the noodles and peas into the bowl with the dressing, along with the clementines, carrots, coriander and cashews. Toss to combine, then serve in bowls or pack into rigid airtight containers to take to work.

Cod puttanesca with spinach & spaghetti

Ingredients

100g wholemeal spaghetti

1 large onion, sliced

1 tbsp rapeseed oil

1 red chilli, deseeded and sliced

2 garlic cloves, chopped

200g cherry tomatoes, halved

1 tsp cider vinegar

2 tsp capers

5 Kalamata olives, halved

½ tsp smoked paprika

2 skinless cod fillet or loins

160g spinach leaves

small handful chopped parsley, to serve

Directions

STEP 1

Boil the spaghetti for 10 mins until al dente, adding the spinach for the last 2 mins. Meanwhile, fry the onion in the oil in a large non-stick frying pan with a lid until tender and turning golden. Stir in the chilli and garlic, then add the tomatoes.

STEP 2

Add the vinegar, capers, olives and paprika with a ladleful of the pasta water. Put the cod fillets on top, then cover the pan and cook for 5-7 mins until the fish just flakes. Drain the pasta and wilted spinach and pile on to plates, then top with the fish and sauce. Sprinkle over some parsley to serve.

WHOLESOME RECIPES FOR DINNER

Moroccan-style vegetable platter

Ingredients

2 tbsp rapeseed oil

2 garlic cloves, finely chopped

2 aubergines (about 500g), sliced

4 tomatoes, cut into wedges

1 tsp ground cumin

10g coriander, chopped

10g parsley, chopped

1 lemon, juiced

8 flatbreads

250g pack cooked beetroot, sliced

2 x 80g packs pomegranate seeds

1 mint sprig (optional)

For the dip

320g frozen baby broad beans

1 tsp cumin seeds

2 large garlic cloves

1 tbsp extra virgin olive oil

1 tsp smoked paprika

Directions

STEP 1

For the dip, boil the broad beans for 7 mins, then drain, reserving the cooking water. Tip into a bowl with the cumin, garlic, oil, paprika and 6 tbsp of the reserved water, then blitz using a hand blender until smooth. Spoon into two small bowls.

STEP 2

Heat the oil in a pan over a medium heat and cook the garlic and aubergines, covered, for 10 mins, stirring occasionally until tender and slightly charred. Add the tomatoes and cumin, and cook for 5-10 mins, then turn off the heat. Add the herbs and lemon juice.

STEP 3

Serve half on a platter with one bowl of dip, four flatbreads and half the beetroot, along with the pomegranate seeds and mint, if using. You can warm the flatbreads in a frying pan or microwave before serving. Chill the remainder to eat cold the next day. Will keep covered and chilled for a day.

Chilli cornbread pie

Ingredients

2 tsp rapeseed oil

2 red onions (320g), finely chopped

2 celery sticks (about 150g), sliced

1 tbsp hot chilli powder

1 tbsp ground coriander

1 tsp ground cumin

3 garlic cloves, finely grated

500g carton passata

2 x 400g cans three bean salad in water

2 tsp gluten-free vegetable bouillon powder

20g coriander, leaves picked and chopped

For the cornbread

50g fine cornmeal

100g gram (chickpea) flour

1 tsp gluten-free baking powder

1 tsp hot chilli powder

1 egg

150ml bio yogurt

50ml milk

50g mature cheddar, coarsely grated

For the corn salad

1 small red onion (about 80g), finely chopped

12 pitted Kalamata olives, roughly chopped

4 tsp balsamic vinegar

2 x 198g cans sweetcorn, drained

1 bag mixed leaf salad

Directions

STEP 1

Heat the oil in a non-stick pan over a medium heat and fry the onions and celery for 8 mins, stirring often. Stir in the spices and garlic, then pour in the passata, bean salad (along with the liquid from the cans) and bouillon. Cover and simmer for 10 mins, then stir in the coriander. Tip into a shallow ovenproof dish and cool slightly.

STEP 2

Heat the oven to 190C/170C fan/ gas 5. Tip the cornmeal, gram flour, baking powder and chilli powder into a bowl and mix well. Beat the egg, yogurt and milk together in a separate bowl, then pour into the dry Ingredients and mix to make a batter. Stir in the cheese, then pour this over the bean chilli and bake for 30-35 mins until the cornbread is puffed up and golden. Combine half the Ingredients for the corn salad and serve with half the chilli, reserving the rest for another day. The pie will keep covered and chilled for four days. Reheat in the microwave until piping hot.

Healthy meatloaf with spaghetti sauce

Ingredients

2 tsp rapeseed oil, plus extra for the dish

320g carrots, finely chopped

2 celery sticks (about 135g), finely chopped

1 onion (about 125g), finely chopped

500g lean 5% fat pork mince

1 egg

25g porridge oats

1 tbsp smoked paprika, plus 1 tsp

30g basil, leaves and stems separated

1½ tsp vegetable bouillon powder

3 large garlic cloves, finely grated

500ml passata

40g mature cheddar, grated

350g wholemeal spaghetti

Directions

STEP 1

Heat the oven to 200C/180C fan/gas 6. Heat the oil in a large non-stick saucepan over a medium heat and cook the carrots, celery and onion, covered, for 10 mins until soft and starting to caramelise. Stir halfway through to prevent burning.

STEP 2

Meanwhile, tip the pork into a bowl with the egg, oats and 1 tbsp smoked paprika. Chop the basil stems and most of the leaves, leaving a few whole. Add the chopped stems and half the chopped leaves to the mixture, along with ½ tsp bouillon. Season with black pepper, then mix with your hands to fully combine. Tip in half the cooked veg, cool for about a minute, then work the veg into the mixture. Shape into a loaf (about 21 x 7cm), then lift into a shallow, lightly oiled baking dish. Brush the top with a little oil as well. Bake for 25 mins until firm.

STEP 3

For the sauce, add the garlic to the remaining veg. Return to a medium heat and cook for 1 min. Stir in the rest of the paprika and bouillon, along with the passata and 100ml water. Cover and simmer for 10 mins. Stir in the remaining chopped basil.

STEP 4

Remove the loaf from the oven and pour over the sauce. Scatter over the cheese, then bake for 10 mins more. Meanwhile, cook the spaghetti following pack instructions. Serve the spaghetti in bowls, topped with the slices of the loaf, a few spoonfuls of sauce and the whole basil leaves.

Tahini noodles with red cabbage & Sichuan peppercorn slaw

Ingredients

½ red cabbage, finely shredded

½ tsp Sichuan peppercorns, toasted and lightly crushed

5g coriander, roughly chopped

1 lime, juiced

3 tbsp tahini

2 garlic cloves, grated

3 tsp low-sodium soy sauce

1 tsp crispy chilli oil, plus extra to serve (optional)

140g dried egg noodles (2 nests)

Directions

STEP 1

Toss the cabbage with the Sichuan peppercorns, coriander and some seasoning. Squeeze over the lime juice, then scrunch it well together. Set aside. Will keep chilled for two days in an airtight container.

STEP 2

Whisk the tahini, garlic, soy sauce and crispy chilli oil together in a large bowl. Cook the noodles in a pan of boiling of salted water following pack instructions until tender. Drain, reserving 125ml of the cooking water. Whisk the reserved water into the tahini sauce, then toss through the noodles.

STEP 3

Divide the noodles between two bowls and top with
the slaw.

Vegan aubergine no-parmigiana

Ingredients

2 tbsp olive oil, plus 2 drops for the baking sheets

3 aubergines, sliced lengthways, about ½cm thick

For the tomato sauce

2 onions, finely chopped

2 garlic cloves, finely grated

800g chopped tomatoes

1 tsp dried oregano

1 tbsp balsamic vinegar

400g can borlotti beans, drained

15g fresh basil leaves, chopped, plus a few for scattering

For the topping

400g can cannellini beans, drained

150ml soya milk

1 tbsp miso paste

30g pine nuts

4 handfuls rocket

Directions

STEP 1

Heat the oven to 200C/180C fan/gas 6. Line two baking sheets with baking parchment, then cover each one lightly with a drop of oil. Press on the aubergine slices, then turn them over so they end up with just a tiny slick of oil on both sides. Roast in the oven for 15-20 mins until tender.

STEP 2

While the aubergines are cooking, make the sauce. Heat the 2 tbsp oil in a pan and fry the onions and garlic over a low heat until softened. Tip in the tomatoes, oregano, balsamic vinegar, borlotti beans and half the basil, then cover and simmer for 15 mins.

STEP 3

To make the topping, put the cannellini beans in a bowl with the soya milk and miso paste, and blitz with a hand blender until smooth.

STEP 4

Cover the base of a large shallow ovenproof dish (about 20cm x 25cm) with half the tomato sauce. Take a third of the aubergine slices, including all of the end pieces – roughly chop the end pieces and arrange over the tomato sauce with the slices. Spread with the rest of the tomato sauce and all of the remaining slices of aubergine to seal in the sauce. Pour over the miso mixture, scatter over the pine nuts, then cover with foil and bake for 40 mins. Uncover then cook for 10 mins more until the topping is set. Scatter with the remaining basil.

Spinach crespolini

Ingredients

50g spelt wholemeal flour

1 egg

100ml milk

½ tsp rapeseed oil

250g baby spinach

generous grating of nutmeg

1 large garlic clove, finely grated

80g ricotta

2 tbsp vegetarian Italian-style hard cheese, finely grated

For the sauce

400g can chopped tomatoes

10g basil

½ tsp vegetable bouillon powder

1 garlic clove, crushed

For the salad

2 tsp balsamic vinegar

1 small red onion (about 80g), finely chopped

80g diced celery

3 handfuls of rocket

160g cherry tomatoes

Directions

STEP 1

Whisk the flour and egg together, then gradually whisk in the milk to create a smooth pancake-style batter. Pour into a jug.

STEP 2

Heat the oil in a 19cm non-stick pan over a medium heat, tip in a quarter of the batter, and swirl to cover the base. Cook briefly until just set, then flip over using a palette knife and cook the other side until just golden. Lift onto a plate, then repeat with the remaining batter to make four pancakes in total.

STEP 3

Meanwhile, heat a second large non-stick pan over a medium heat and cook the spinach, nutmeg and garlic for about 5 mins, stirring with a wooden spoon until the spinach has completely wilted. Remove from the heat and cool slightly, then beat in the ricotta. Spoon a quarter of the spinach filling down the centre of each pancake, then roll up into a sausage and arrange snugly in an ovenproof dish. Heat the oven to 200C/180C fan/gas 6.

STEP 4

To make the sauce, put the canned tomatoes, basil, bouillon and garlic in a bowl, and blitz using a hand blender until completely smooth (or do this in a jug blender). Pour the sauce over the pancakes and scatter over the cheese. Bake for 30 mins until browned and bubbling at the edges. For the salad, combine the vinegar, onion and celery. Just before serving, toss the onion mixture with the rocket and tomatoes, and serve with the filled pancakes.

Courgette curry with lemon rice

Ingredients

For the curry

1 tbsp olive oil

2 tbsp ginger, very finely chopped

1½ tsp cumin seeds

1-2 red chillies, deseeded and finely chopped

6 garlic cloves, crushed

450g baby potatoes, thickly sliced

2 tsp ground coriander

1 tsp ground turmeric

4 large vine tomatoes, roughly chopped

1 tbsp tomato purée

200ml stock, made with 1 tsp vegetable bouillon powder

1 cinnamon stick

500g medium-sized courgettes, thickly sliced

15g chopped fresh coriander

For the lemon rice

1 tbsp olive oil

½-1 tsp brown mustard seeds (optional)

240g brown basmati rice

½-1 tsp turmeric

12 curry leaves (optional)

400g can chickpeas, drained

2 tbsp lemon juice

Directions

STEP 1

Heat the oil in a large frying pan and fry the ginger for 3 mins. Stir in the cumin seeds, chillies and garlic and cook briefly, then add the potatoes, ground coriander and turmeric, and stir well. Tip in the tomatoes, tomato purée and stock, then add the cinnamon, cover, and leave to simmer for 5 mins.

STEP 2

Stir in the courgettes, then cover and cook for 10-12 mins until the courgettes are tender rather than soft. Stir in the fresh coriander.

STEP 3

Meanwhile, heat the oil in a pan and stir in the mustard seeds, if using, and cook until you hear them pop. Stir in the rice, turmeric and curry leaves, if using, then pour in 1 litre boiling water. Simmer, covered, for 15 mins, then add the chickpeas and lemon juice, cover once again, and cook for 10 mins more until the water has been absorbed and the rice is tender.

Portobello jackfruit burgers

Ingredients

900g potatoes, cut into slim chips

3 tbsp rapeseed oil, plus a drop

8 large flat portobello mushrooms (600g), stalks removed

smoked paprika, for sprinkling

For the burgers

410g can jackfruit in water, drained

2 tsp tamari

400g chickpeas, well drained

1 tbsp tomato purée

2 garlic cloves, chopped

2 tbsp wholemeal spelt flour

For the tomato relish

4 vine tomatoes, finely chopped

2 tsp tomato purée

1 tsp balsamic vinegar

2 tbsp finely chopped red onion

1-2 tbsp chopped basil or coriander

Directions

STEP 1

Heat the oven to 200C/180C fan/gas 6. Toss the chips in 2½ tbsp of the oil and spread out on a large non-stick baking sheet lined with baking parchment. Rub the outside of the mushrooms with a drop of oil, then arrange them on another baking sheet, rounded-side up, and put the chips and mushrooms in the oven for 20 mins. Turn the mushrooms and chips over after 10 mins.

STEP 2

Meanwhile, squeeze as much juice as you can out of the jackfruit. The best way is to wrap it in kitchen paper, then squeeze with your hands. Trim off the feathery bits of jackfruit that look a bit like shredded meat, weigh out 75g and stir in the tamari sauce. Tip the remaining jackfruit into a bowl. Add the chickpeas, tomato purée and garlic and blitz together until smooth using a hand blender or use a food processor. Stir in the remaining jackfruit and shape into four burgers about the size of the mushrooms. Coat in the flour.

STEP 3

Check the chips and mushrooms and cook for 5-10 mins longer if needed. Meanwhile, heat the remaining oil and fry two of the burgers for a few minutes each side until brown and heated through. To make the relish, put the chopped tomatoes in a bowl with the tomato purée, vinegar, onion and basil or coriander.

STEP 4

To serve, sandwich two of the burgers between the mushrooms. If the mushrooms are very juicy, blot with a little kitchen paper first. Serve with half the chips, sprinkled with the paprika, and serve half the relish on the side. The remaining mushrooms, burgers and chips will keep for two days in the fridge. To serve again, warm the remaining mushrooms and burgers in a low oven, and heat the chips, uncovered, until piping hot.

Spicy chickpea stew

Ingredients

1 tbsp rapeseed oil

2 onions (320g), roughly chopped

2 green peppers, deseeded and cut into cubes

2 tsp hot chilli powder

1 tbsp ground coriander

1 tsp ground cumin

500ml carton passata

2 x 400g cans chickpeas

2 tsp vegetable bouillon powder

40g flame raisins

½ lemon, juiced, flesh scooped out and white pith removed, then zest finely chopped (you'll need 2 tsp)

350g cauliflower florets

15g parsley, chopped

140g wholemeal couscous

40g toasted flaked almonds

Directions

STEP 1

Heat the oil in a large lidded pan over a medium heat and fry the onions for 10 mins, stirring often until golden. Stir in the peppers and cook for 5 mins more.

STEP 2

Add the chilli powder, coriander and cumin, stir briefly, then tip in the passata and chickpeas along with the liquid from the cans.

STEP 3

Stir in the bouillon powder, raisins and lemon zest, then add the cauliflower. Cover tightly and simmer over a medium heat for 15-20 mins until the cauliflower is tender. Stir in half the parsley.

STEP 4

Meanwhile, put the couscous in a heatproof bowl and pour over 175ml boiling water from the kettle. Stir in the lemon juice, then cover and let stand for about 10 mins until the couscous has absorbed the liquid and is tender. Stir in the toasted flaked almonds and most of the remaining parsley.

STEP 5

Divide half the couscous between two plates and top with half the chickpea stew and the rest of the parsley. Leave the remainder to cool for another day. Will keep covered and chilled for up to three days. Reheat the stew in a pan over a low heat with a splash of water until piping hot. Reheat the couscous in the microwave.

Air fryer roast dinner

Ingredients

2-3 medium potatoes, peeled and cut into quarters

3 tsp vegetable, olive or rapeseed oil

1 large or 2 small chicken breasts, skin-on

3 medium carrots, peeled and cut into batons

100g frozen peas

gravy, to serve

Directions

STEP 1

Soak the potatoes in water for 30 mins, then drain and rinse. Heat the air fryer for 2 mins. Dry the potatoes thoroughly, then put in a bowl, drizzle over 1 tsp of the oil and season with salt and pepper. Using your hands or a spoon, coat the potatoes in the oil, then put into the air fryer basket, in one layer if possible. Cook for 10 mins at 190C.

STEP 2

Meanwhile, coat the chicken in another 1 tsp oil and season with salt and freshly ground black pepper. Once the potatoes have been in for 10 mins, move them to the sides and lay the chicken in the centre of the basket. Cook for 10 mins.

STEP 3

Coat the carrots in the remaining oil. After the chicken has cooked for 10 mins, remove it from the basket and add the carrots, mixed in with the potatoes, then move both to the sides and put the chicken back into the centre. Cook for 10-15 mins, still at 190C. At this point, the chicken should be cooked – check by inserting a knife into the thickest part and checking the juices run clear. Alternatively, a meat thermometer should read 70C. If it's not quite done, cook for a further 5 mins. Remove the chicken and rest it under a piece of tented foil.

STEP 4

Put the peas in a small ovenproof dish or mug with 2 tbsp water and cover with foil to prevent any moisture escaping. Put in the air fryer basket where the chicken was and cook for a final 10 mins at 190C. The potatoes should be golden and crisp, the carrots tender and the peas warmed through. Slice the chicken breast and serve with the vegetables and gravy.

Giant couscous salad with charred veg & tangy pesto

Ingredients

2-3 raw beetroot (320g), peeled and chopped

3 red onions (320g), cut into wedges

2 green or orange peppers, deseeded and cubed

1 tbsp olive oil

320g cherry tomatoes

200g wholewheat giant couscous

For the pesto

7g fresh coriander, roughly chopped

15g flat-leaf parsley, roughly chopped

1 garlic clove

1 green chilli, deseeded

½ tsp cumin

1 tbsp apple cider vinegar

1 tbsp olive oil

40g pine nuts, lightly toasted

Directions

STEP 1

Heat the oven to 200C/180C fan/gas 6. In a bowl, toss the beetroot, onions and peppers together with the oil, then spread out on a large roasting tray lined with baking paper and roast for 35 mins. Scatter over the cherry tomatoes, then return to the oven for 10 mins more until the tomatoes have softened and the vegetables are tender.

STEP 2

Meanwhile, cook the couscous following pack instructions, then rinse and drain. To make the pesto, put the coriander and half the parsley in a bowl with the garlic, chilli, cumin, vinegar, oil and 25g of the pine nuts. Add 2 tbsp water, then blitz with a hand blender until smooth or use a small food processor.

STEP 3

Toss the roasted veg and chopped parsley through the couscous and pile on the pesto, then scatter with the remaining pine nuts.

Healthy pad Thai

100g brown rice flat noodles

1 tbsp rapeseed oil

2 skinless chicken thigh fillets, chopped

1 onion (160g), roughly chopped

1 red pepper, deseeded and cut into thin slices

1 small carrot (60g), peeled into thick ribbons using a veg peeler

3 garlic cloves, sliced

1 red chilli, deseeded and thinly sliced

1 tbsp finely grated ginger

100g beansprouts

15g roasted unsalted peanuts

2 tbsp lime juice, plus 1 tsp zest

1 tbsp low-salt soy sauce

15g chopped coriander

handful of chopped basil

Directions

STEP 1

Tip the noodles into a bowl and soak following pack instructions until tender but not soft – you don't want them to become mushy. Drain.

STEP 2

Heat the oil in a wok over a medium-high heat and stir-fry the chicken for 5 mins until cooked. Transfer the chicken to a bowl and set aside, keeping the oil in the wok. Stir-fry the onion, pepper and carrot for 5 mins to soften, then add the garlic, chilli and ginger, and cook for a few minutes more until fragrant.

STEP 3

Add the beansprouts, turn up the heat to high, and stir through the peanuts, lime juice and zest and the soy sauce. Return the chicken to the pan along with the noodles and herbs, and gently toss everything together until heated through. Best served straightaway.

One-pot five-spice rice

Ingredients

1 tbsp rapeseed oil

2 garlic cloves, thinly sliced

25g ginger, peeled and finely shredded

½-1 tsp Chinese five-spice powder

1 fresh chilli, deseeded and sliced

2 red peppers, deseeded and diced

200g easy-cook brown rice

650ml vegetable stock, made with 2 tsp bouillon
powder

420g frozen mixed beans (broad beans, peas and French beans)

½ pack spring onions, (about 8), trimmed and sliced

2 tsp sesame oil

75g roasted cashews

Directions

STEP 1

Heat the rapeseed oil in a large pan over a medium heat and fry the garlic and ginger for 5 mins. Add the five-spice, chilli, peppers and rice, then pour in the stock, cover tightly and cook for 15 mins.

STEP 2

Stir in the frozen beans and spring onions, then cover and cook for 10 mins. Check the rice is tender; if not, leave for 5 mins more. Turn off the heat, stir in the sesame oil and leave to stand, covered, for 5 mins.

STEP 3

Divide the rice between two bowls and scatter over half the cashews. Leave the remainder to cool completely for another day. Will keep chilled in an airtight container for up to three days. Reheat in a microwave until piping hot, then add the cashews.

WHOLESOME RECIPES FOR SNACK

Avocado & strawberry ices

Ingredients

200g ripe strawberries, hulled and chopped

1 avocado, stoned, peeled and roughly chopped

2 tsp balsamic vinegar

½ tsp vanilla extract

1-2 tsp maple syrup (optional)

Directions

STEP 1

Put the strawberries (save four pieces for the top),
avocado, vinegar and vanilla in a bowl and blitz
using a hand blender (or in a food processor) until
as smooth as you can get it. Have a taste and only
add the maple syrup if the strawberries are not
sweet enough.

STEP 2

Pour into containers, add a strawberry to each,
cover with cling film and freeze. Allow the pots to
soften for 5-10 mins before eating.

Microwave butternut squash risotto

Ingredients

250g risotto rice

700ml hot vegetable stock

1 medium butternut squash

big handful grated parmesan (or vegetarian alternative), plus extra

handful sage leaves, roughly chopped

Directions

STEP 1

Tip the rice into a large bowl, then add 500ml of the hot vegetable stock. Cover with cling film and microwave on High for 5 mins. Meanwhile, peel and cut the squash into medium chunks (see tip, below). Stir the rice, then add the squash and the rest of the stock. Re-cover with cling film, then microwave for another 15 mins, stirring halfway, until almost all the stock is absorbed and the rice and squash are tender.

STEP 2

Leave the risotto to sit for 2 mins, then stir in the parmesan and sage. Serve topped with more grated cheese

Pitta pocket

Ingredients

½ wholemeal pitta bread

25g cooked skinless chicken breast

¼ cucumber, cut into chunks

4 cherry tomatoes, halved

Directions

STEP 1

Fill the pitta half with the chicken breast, cucumber and cherry tomatoes.

Mild chilli & bean pasta bake

Ingredients

1 large onion, chopped

2 sticks celery, thinly sliced

340g extra-lean minced beef

2 tsp mild chilli powder

410g can chopped tomatoes

1 tbsp tomato purée

400g can kidney bean in water, drained and rinsed

300ml beef or chicken stock

300g wholewheat penne

For the topping

½ x 568g tub 0% fat Greek yogurt

2 eggs, beaten

50g red leicester cheese, coarsely grated

1 small garlic clove, crushed

Directions

STEP 1

Heat a splash of oil in a frying pan, add the onion and celery, season with pepper and a little salt, then cook until soft. Remove vegetables and set aside. Brown the mince in the pan, a handful at a time, tossing with a fork as you go. Only add a splash of oil if the mixture begins to stick too much. Once browned, tip into a sieve to remove any excess fat.

STEP 2

Return mince and cooked veg to the frying pan, add the chilli powder, tomatoes, tomato purée, beans and stock, bring to the boil and simmer for 15 mins.

STEP 3

Heat oven to 200C/fan 180C/gas 6. Cook the pasta according to pack instructions. Drain, stir into the mince and spoon into a large lasagne dish. Mix the yogurt, eggs, cheese and garlic together and season lightly. Spoon over the top of the pasta and bake for 20-25 mins or until lightly browned.

Sesame flatbreads

Ingredients

200g self-raising flour

2 tbsp sesame seeds

a pinch of salt

a grind of black pepper

150g pot natural yogurt

1 tbsp milk or water

a little olive oil

Directions

STEP 1

Heat grill to high and dust a non-stick baking sheet with a little flour. Mix the self-raising flour, sesame seeds, a pinch of salt and a grind of black pepper in a large bowl. Stir in the natural yogurt and milk or water, then mix well to form a soft dough.

STEP 2

Divide the dough into 4 and press each piece into an oval approx 5mm thick. Place on the sheet and grill for 3 mins on each side until puffed and golden. Brush with a little olive oil before serving, if you like.

Flowerpot bread

Ingredients

500g granary, strong, wholemeal or white bread flour

7g sachet fast-action dried yeast

1 tsp salt

2 tbsp olive oil, plus extra for the flowerpots

1 tbsp clear honey

a little milk or oil, for brushing

Plus any of these toppings

1 tbsp pumpkin, sunflower, sesame or poppy seed

4 tbsp grated cheddar or crumbled feta cheese

1 tbsp chopped rosemary, thyme, oregano, chives
or basil

1 tbsp chopped olive or sundried tomatoes

½ tsp chilli flakes

You will also need

5 small, clean clay flowerpots (see tip below),
baking parchment and cling film

Directions

STEP 1

Tip the flour, yeast and salt into a large bowl. Pour
in 300ml warm water, the olive oil and honey. Mix
with a wooden spoon until the mixture clumps

together, then tip out onto a work surface. Use your hands to stretch and knead the dough for about 10 mins, or until it's smooth and springy. Add a little extra flour if the dough feels too sticky.

STEP 2

Brush the flowerpots with oil and line the sides with baking parchment. Divide the dough into 5 pieces and shape into smooth balls. Place one ball of dough into each flowerpot and cover with cling film. Leave in a warm place for 1 hr to rise.

STEP 3

Heat oven to 200C/180C fan/gas 6. When the dough has doubled in size, remove the cling film from the pots and gently brush with a little milk or oil. Sprinkle with your choice of topping.

STEP 4

Place the pots on a baking tray in the oven and cook for 20-25 mins until risen and golden. The pots will be very hot, so be careful when removing from the oven. Leave to cool for 10 mins before turning out and eating.

Healthy veg patch hummus

Ingredients

1 x 400g can chickpeas, drained and rinsed

½ lemon, juiced

1 garlic clove, crushed

2 tbsp olive oil

2 tbsp tahini

250g baby carrots

1 pot of parsley

Directions

STEP 1

Put the chickpeas, lemon juice, garlic, olive oil and tahini into a food processor and blitz to a smooth consistency. Loosen with 1–2 tbsp water if it seems a little thick.

STEP 2

Make a hole in the top of each carrot with a skewer or by cutting a small hole with the tip of a sharp knife. Dab a small amount of hummus into the hole and push in a small sprig of parsley.

STEP 3

Spoon the hummus into thoroughly cleaned small, plant pots or bowls and push in the carrots. Let the children dunk into the hummus with the carrots.

Peppery fennel & carrot salad

Ingredients

2 large carrots, cut into thin sticks or grated

2 large fennel bulbs, quartered and thinly sliced

handful peanut or cashew nuts, chopped

2 tbsp olive oil

1 tsp mustard seed

1 tsp nigella or black onion seeds (optional)

juice 1 lemon or lime

Directions

STEP 1

Tip the carrots and fennel into a salad bowl. Toast the nuts in a hot frying pan for 3-5 mins until golden, then tip onto a plate. In the same pan, heat the oil and fry the mustard and nigella or black onion seeds, if using, until they begin to pop – about 30 secs. Pour in the lemon or lime juice and mix together to make a dressing. Toss together with the vegetables in the bowl, then sprinkle with nuts to serve.

Couscous with pine nuts, coriander & raisins

Ingredients

250g couscous

400ml hot vegetable stock

75g 2 ½ oz pine nuts

50g dried apricots, chopped

bunch coriander leaves

4-5 tbsp raisins

zest and juice 1 lemon

5 tbsp olive oil

Directions

STEP 1

Put the couscous in a medium-sized bowl, pour over the stock, cover with cling film, and leave to stand for 5 mins. Meanwhile, toast the pine nuts in a dry pan for a few mins, until pale golden.

STEP 2

Fluff up the couscous with a fork, add all the remaining Ingredients and mix well to combine.

Spicy chicken with mango salad

Ingredients

4 skinless boneless chicken breasts

drizzle olive oil

1 tbsp garam masala

1 large ripe mango

½ cucumber

½ small red onion

handful fresh coriander leaves

4 tbsp soured cream or natural yogurt

grated zest and juice ½ lime

warm naan bread, to serve

Directions

STEP 1

Heat a griddle or frying pan until hot. Rub the chicken with oil, garam masala and a good pinch of salt. Cook for 6 minutes on each side or until slightly charred and cooked through.

STEP 2

Peel and slice the mango into slim wedges. Halve the cucumber lengthways and slice thickly at an angle. Thinly slice the onion. Toss the salad Ingredients together with the coriander and pile onto plates.

STEP 3

Mix the soured cream or yogurt with the lime zest and juice, season and dollop beside the salad. Cut the chicken in half or into thirds diagonally, arrange next to the salad and serve with naan bread.

Stuffed cocktail eggs

Ingredients

12 medium eggs

6 tbsp bio yogurt

2 tsp English mustard

2 tbsp finely chopped parsley

For the salmon eggs

50g smoked salmon

sprigs of fresh dill

For the chorizo crumb eggs

25g chorizo, skin removed and finely chopped

Directions

STEP 1

Boil the eggs for 7 mins, drain and put into iced water to cool. Carefully remove the shells, then cut in half lengthways. Scoop the yolks into a bowl and mash with the yogurt, mustard and parsley. Spoon the mixture back into the eggs.

STEP 2

For the salmon eggs, top each with a strip of salmon and snip over some fresh dill.

STEP 3

For the chorizo version, fry the chorizo gently in a non-stick pan until the oil runs out and the chorizo is crisp. Scatter over the eggs when cool. Keep chilled until ready to serve. Will keep in the fridge for up to one day.

Peanut hummus with fruit & veg sticks

Ingredients

380g carton chickpeas

zest and juice 0.5 lemon (use the other 1/2 to squeeze over the apple to stop it browning, if you like)

1 tbsp tahini

0.5-1 tsp smoked paprika

2 tbsp roasted unsalted peanuts

1 tsp rapeseed oil

2 crisp red apples, cored and cut into slices

2 carrots, cut into sticks

4 celery sticks, cut into batons lengthways

Directions

STEP 1

Drain the chickpeas, reserving the liquid. Tip three-quarters of the chickpeas into a food processor and add the lemon zest and juice, tahini, paprika, peanuts and oil with 3 tbsp chickpea liquid. Blitz in a food processor until smooth, then stir in the reserved chickpeas. Serve with the fruit and veg sticks.

Healthy Easter boiled eggs

Ingredients

6 medium eggs

1 tbsp currants

1 small carrot, peeled and cut in to small triangles

80g cherry tomatoes

80g sliced cucumber

30g rocket

A few sprigs of rosemary, to serve

Mini carrots, to serve

Directions

STEP 1

Bring a large pan of water to the boil. Add the eggs and simmer for 10 mins. Drain the eggs and plunge into ice water to cool down, gently peel off the shells and discard.

STEP 2

Cut some of the eggs in half and decorate with currants for eyes and a small triangle of carrot for a beak to create egg chicks (as per picture). Slice the remaining eggs to create bunny shapes (as per picture) quartering some for ears and halving some lengthways for the body. Create a round tail by slicing the top off one of the eggs.

STEP 3

Decorate the plate/board with sprigs of rosemary and miniature carrots, if you like. Serve with the cucumber, cherry tomatoes and rocket.

Crispy roasted chickpeas

Ingredients

1 x 400g can chickpeas, drained

1tsp rapeseed oil

2tsp smoked paprika

2tsp ground cumin

2tsp ground coriander

½tsp cayenne pepper

Directions

STEP 1

Heat oven to 200C/180C fan/gas 4. Tip the chickpeas into a bowl and toss with the rapeseed oil, smoked paprika, cumin and coriander along with a big pinch of salt. Toss well until the chickpeas are well coated, then tip out onto a baking tray and bake for 35 mins, moving them round the tray halfway through so they dry out evenly and are crunchy. Leave to cool, then store in an airtight container.

SECTION 5: IN SUMMARY

There isn't a universal dietary plan for managing Barrett's esophagus. Nonetheless, embracing a diet abundant in fruits, vegetables, whole grains, and lean proteins, while limiting fatty and acidic foods, might alleviate symptoms and lower the likelihood of complications.

It's important to note that individuals may react differently to certain foods, underscoring the necessity for patients to collaborate closely with healthcare providers to customize dietary advice according to their specific requirements and tastes.

Ultimately, maintaining a well-rounded diet alongside other suggested lifestyle adjustments and medical treatments can greatly contribute to promoting overall health and effectively managing Barrett's esophagus.